Copyright 2023

All right reserved.No part of this book should be reproduced without express permission of the author.

Reproduction of all or any part of this book is punishable unders relevant law.

Table of Contents

PREVIEW 4

AUTOIMMUNE HEPATITIS DIET RECIPES 5

BREAKFAST 5

   1. Oatmeal Pancakes with Cinnamon Apples 5

   2. This Is the Best Paleo Muffins Recipe 8

   3. Homemade Cranberry-Orange Granola Recipe 10

   4. Instant Pot Zuppa Toscana 12

   5. A Flavor-Packed, Warm Kale-Quinoa Salad 14

   6. Instant Pot Chicken and Rice Soup 16

   7. Copycat Wendy's Chili 19

   8. Copycat Olive Garden Pasta Fagioli 21

   9. Chili Pumpkin 23

   10. Warm Goat Cheese Salad 25

LUNCH 28

   11. Hot Ham and Cheese Sandwich with Chipotle Mayo 28

   12. Classic Herb Roast Chicken with Root Vegetables 31

   13. Easy Cinnamon-Roasted Sweet Potato Salad with Wild Rice 34

   14. Hearty Crock-Pot Beef Ragu 36

   15. Curry with Cauliflower and Butternut Squash Stir Fry 38

16. Orecchiette with Broccoli Rabe 41

17. The Best-Ever Healthy Lasagna 43

18. Healthier Chicken Pot Pie 46

19. Beef Stew in Red Wine 49

20. Turkey Meatloaf 52

DINNERS 55

21. Creamy Mushroom Chicken 55

22. Zucchini Carbonara with Bacon 58

23. Flavorful Basque Chicken 60

24. Spicy Macaroni and Cheese with Jalapeños and Prosciutto 62

25. Paleo Turkey Bolognese with Garlic Spaghetti Squash 65

26. Tandoori Chicken Legs and Roasted Cauliflower 68

27. Pumpkin Version of Pad Thai 70

28. Paleo BBQ Pork Shepherd's Pie with Sweet Potato Topping 72

29. Low-Calorie Braised Brisket with Horseradish 74

30. Easy Chicken and Dumplings 77

PREVIEW

Autoimmune hepatitis is liver inflammation that occurs when your body's immune system turns against liver cells. The exact cause of autoimmune hepatitis is unclear, but genetic and environmental factors appear to interact over time in triggering the disease.

Untreated autoimmune hepatitis can lead to scarring of the liver (cirrhosis) and eventually to liver failure. When diagnosed and treated early, however, autoimmune hepatitis often can be controlled with drugs that suppress the immune system.

A liver transplant may be an option when autoimmune hepatitis doesn't respond to drug treatments or in cases of advanced liver disease.

AUTOIMMUNE HEPATITIS DIET RECIPES

BREAKFAST

1. Oatmeal Pancakes with Cinnamon Apples

Prep Time: 25 Minutes

Cook Time: 50 Minutes

Serves: 4

Ingredients

- 1 1/2 cups buttermilk
- 3/4 cup instant rolled oats
- 3/4 cup whole wheat flour
- 2 Tbsp milk
- 1 Tbsp melted butter
- 1 1/2 tsp baking powder
- 1/2 tsp baking soda
- Pinch of cinnamon (plus 1/8 tsp for the apples)

- Pinch of nutmeg
- 1 Granny Smith apple, peeled, cored, and chopped
- ½ cup apple juice
- 2 Tbsp brown sugar
- Butter or cooking spray
- Confectioners' sugar

Instructions

1. In a large mixing bowl, combine the buttermilk, oats, flour, milk, butter, baking powder, baking soda, pinch of cinnamon, and nutmeg. Stir to gently combine, then set aside to rest for a few minutes.
2. Combine the apple, apple juice, brown sugar, and remaining ⅛ teaspoon cinnamon in a small saucepan and bring to a simmer. Cook until the apple has softened and the liquid has thickened.
3. Preheat the oven to 200°F. Heat a large nonstick or cast-iron skillet over medium heat. Adding a bit of butter or cooking spray before each round, scoop ¼-cup portions of batter into the skillet and use a spatula to spread into thin, even circles. Cook until small bubbles form in the top of the batter, 2 to 3 minutes, then flip and cook for another 2 minutes. Keep

pancakes warm in the oven while you finish cooking. Serve topped with the warm apples and a bit of confectioners' sugar, if you like.

Eat This Tip

1. Fret not, for all of these fruit toppings are not only better for you than normal syrup, they're also considerably more exciting. Combine in a small saucepan and simmer for 10 minutes:

- 2 cups frozen (or fresh) blueberries, 2 tablespoons sugar, and 1 tablespoon grated ginger
- 2 cups frozen strawberries, 1 tablespoon sugar, and 2 tablespoons balsamic vinegar
- 2 cups diced pineapple simmered in 1 cup lite coconut milk and 2 Tbsp shredded coconut

2. This Is the Best Paleo Muffins Recipe

Prep Time: 15 Minutes

Cook Time: 50 Minutes

Serves: 12

Ingredients

- 3 eggs
- ½ cup coconut sugar, plus extra for sprinkling
- ⅓ cup melted and slightly cooled coconut oil
- ⅓ cup olive oil
- 2 teaspoons orange zest
- 2 tablespoons ground flaxseed
- 1 teaspoon vanilla extract
- 1 ½ cups almond flour
- ½ cup coconut flour
- 2 teaspoons baking powder
- 1 teaspoon kosher salt
- 1 teaspoon cinnamon
- 6 small plums or pluots, pitted and quartered

Instructions

1. Preheat oven to 350°F. Line a 12-cup muffin pan with cupcake liners or grease with nonstick cooking spray.
2. In a medium bowl, whisk together eggs, coconut sugar, coconut oil, olive oil, orange zest, flaxseed, and vanilla.
3. Whisk in almond flour, coconut flour, baking powder, salt, and cinnamon.
4. Evenly divide batter among muffin cups.
5. Press 2 plum slices into the center of each muffin and sprinkle with more coconut sugar.
6. Bake for 30-35 minutes, or until a toothpick stuck into the center of a muffin comes out clean. Store in airtight containers at room temperature or in the refrigerator for about 1 week, or in the freezer for 2 months.

3. Homemade Cranberry-Orange Granola Recipe

Prep Time: 10 Minutes

Cook Time: 30 Minutes

Serves: 10

Ingredients

- Nonstick cooking spray
- 2 1/2 cups regular rolled oats
- 1 cup wheat flakes
- 1/3 cup whole bran cereal such as Grape-Nuts
- 1/3 cup coarsely chopped pecans
- 1/2 cup orange juice
- 2 Tbsp pure maple syrup
- 2 tsp orange zest
- 1/2 tsp pumpkin pie spice
- 1/2 cup dried cranberries
- Fat-free milk, nonfat yogurt, or fresh fruit (optional)

Instructions

1. Preheat oven to 325°F. Coat a 15 x 10 x 1-inch pan with nonstick cooking spray or line with parchment paper; set aside.
2. In a large bowl, stir together oats, wheat flakes, bran cereal, and pecans. In a small saucepan, stir together orange juice, maple syrup, orange zest, and pumpkin pie spice. Cook and stir just until boiling. Remove from heat. Pour over oat mixture; toss just until coated.
3. Spread oat mixture evenly in prepared pan. Bake for 30 to 35 minutes, or until oats are lightly browned, stirring twice. Remove from oven and stir in dried cranberries.
4. Immediately turn out onto a large piece of foil; cool completely. Serve with milk or use to make a breakfast parfait with nonfat yogurt and fresh fruit.
5. Store in an airtight container in the refrigerator for up to 2 weeks or in the freezer for up to 3 months.
6. Not all granolas are created equal. Many store-bought varieties are loaded with added sugars and fat. Whip up this homemade version to save calories without sacrificing flavor.

4. Instant Pot Zuppa Toscana

Prep Time: 10 Minutes

Cook Time: 30 Minutes

Serves: 5

Ingredients

- 1 lb. spicy Italian sausage, ground
- 4 slices bacon, diced
- 1 onion, diced
- 2 garlic cloves, minced
- 4 cups chicken stock
- 4 russet potatoes, peeled and diced
- 4 cups of kale, loosely packed
- 1 cup light cream
- Salt and pepper
- Red pepper flakes

Instructions

1. Turn on the Sauté feature of the Instant Pot. Add 1 tsp of olive oil, the ground Italian sausage, and the bacon slices. Cook for about 3 minutes.

2. Add in the onion and garlic cloves. Saute for another 3 minutes, or until the sausage has browned.
3. Add in the russet potatoes and chicken stock. Seal the lid and cook on high pressure (Manual/High Pressure) for 10 minutes. Release the pressure immediately.
4. Turn the Sauté feature back on.
5. Add the kale and the heavy cream. Stir until warmed through and the kale has wilted (another 3 to 5 minutes). Sprinkle in salt and pepper to taste.
6. Serve with red pepper flakes sprinkled on top and fresh parmesan cheese, if desired.

5. A Flavor-Packed, Warm Kale-Quinoa Salad

Prep Time: 10 Minutes

Cook Time: 30 Minutes

Serves: 4

Ingredients

- 1 medium sweet potato
- 2 Tbsp olive oil, divided
- 1/8 tsp salt
- 1 1/2 cups reduced-sodium chicken broth
- 3/4 cup dry quinoa, rinsed and drained
- 1/2 cup thin wedges red onion
- 6 cups coarsely torn, trimmed kale
- 2 cups coarsely shredded, cooked chicken
- 1 medium apple, quartered, cored, and thinly sliced
- 1 recipe Dijon Vinaigrette (recipe below)
- 1/2 cup coarsely chopped walnuts or pecans (toasted)

Instructions

1. Preheat oven to 425°F. Peel sweet potato. Cut into quarters lengthwise; thinly slice quarters crosswise.

Arrange potato slices in a shallow baking pan. Drizzle with 1 Tbsp of the oil; sprinkle with salt. Toss potatoes to coat. Roast, uncovered, for 15 to 20 minutes or until potatoes are just tender, stirring once halfway through roasting.
2. Meanwhile, in a large skillet, heat broth and quinoa to boiling; reduce heat. Simmer, covered, for 12 to 15 minutes or until quinoa is tender and most of the liquid is absorbed. Drain if needed; transfer quinoa to a bowl. Cover to keep warm.
3. In the same skillet, heat remaining 1 Tbsp oil over medium heat. Add onion; cook for 4 to 5 minutes or until onion is starting to soften, stirring occasionally. Add kale. Cook for 2 to 3 minutes more or until kale is just wilted, tossing frequently with tongs.
4. Immediately divide kale mixture among four shallow serving bowls. Top kale with cooked quinoa, sweet potato, chicken, and apple. Drizzle with dijon vinaigrette (recipe below). Sprinkle with walnuts.

How to Make Dijon Vinaigrette
1. In a small screw-top jar, add 3 Tbsp cider vinegar, 1/3 cup olive oil, 2 tsp Dijon mustard, 1/2 teaspoon dried thyme, and 1/4 teaspoon salt. Cover; shake well until fully combined.

6. Instant Pot Chicken and Rice Soup

Prep Time: 25 Minutes

Cook Time: 55 Minutes

Serves: 8

Ingredients

- 2 garlic cloves, minced
- 1 yellow onion, diced
- 3 carrots, diced
- 2 celery stalks, diced
- 1 lb. chicken breast
- 5 cups chicken broth
- 1 cup wild rice
- 1/2 tsp dried thyme
- 2 bay leaves
- 1/2 tsp salt
- 1/4 tsp pepper
- 1/4 cup unbleached all-purpose flour
- 1 cup milk
- 5 Tbsp butter

Instructions

2. Turn the Sauté feature on the Instant Pot. Once hot, melt 1 tablespoon of butter in the pot. Add the diced onion, minced garlic, carrots, and celery. Cook for three minutes.
3. Add in the chicken breast, chicken broth, wild rice, dried thyme, and the bay leaves. Sprinkle in the salt and pepper, then seal the lid of the Instant Pot.
4. Switch to high pressure (Manual/Pressure Cook) for 20 minutes.
5. When the Instant Pot timer goes off, let it depressurize by itself for 10 minutes. Once finished, release the rest of the pressure from the valve.
6. While the soup is cooking, make a roux on the stove. Melt the other 4 tablespoons of butter in a saucepan.
7. Once melted, sprinkle in the flour and whisk continuously for one minute.
8. When the flour is browned, pour in the milk slowly. Whisk continuously until a thick sauce (a roux) has formed.
9. Remove the bay leaves with tongs from the Instant Pot.
10. Remove the chicken to a cutting board and shred with two forks.

11. Switch it back to the Sauté feature. Pour in the roux into the Instant Pot, then the shredded chicken. Stir until the roux has broken up and a thick soup has formed.

7. Copycat Wendy's Chili

Prep Time: 25 Minutes

Cook Time: 55 Minutes

Serves: 8

Ingredients

- 1 garlic clove, minced
- 1 tablespoon olive oil
- 1 medium onion, diced
- 2 celery stalks, diced
- 1 green bell pepper, diced
- 1 lb. ground beef
- 1 tablespoon taco seasoning
- 1 10 oz can. pinto beans
- 1 10 oz. can kidney beans
- 1 10 oz. can tomato sauce
- 1 10 oz. can diced tomatoes
- Shredded cheddar cheese, for topping
- Sour cream, for topping

Instructions

1. Heat up a dutch oven or a stockpot over medium heat. Add in the olive oil, minced garlic, onion, celery, and

green bell pepper. When the vegetables start to become soft (about three minutes), add in the ground beef.

2. Using a wooden spoon, break up the ground beef and stir in with the vegetables. When the ground beef is no longer pink, using a spoon, drain the grease into an excess can.

3. Add in the beans, tomato sauce, and diced tomatoes into the dutch oven. Sprinkle in the taco seasoning and mix together.

4. Turn the chili on simmer, and let it cook for at least 30 minutes, stirring once in a while so nothing burns at the bottom. The longer you let it sit, the better the flavors will become.

5. Serve with shredded cheese and sour cream, if desired.

8. Copycat Olive Garden Pasta Fagioli

Prep Time: 10 Minutes

Cook Time: 45 Minutes

Serves: 8

Ingredients

- 1 pound ground beef
- 1 yellow onion, diced
- 4 garlic cloves, minced
- 3 carrots, peeled & diced
- 2 celery stalks, diced
- 1 15 oz. can kidney beans, drained
- 1 15 oz. can white (cannellini) beans, drained
- 2 15 oz. can tomato sauce
- 1 15 oz. can diced tomatoes
- 3 cups chicken broth
- 1 tsp dried oregano
- 1 tsp dried thyme leaves
- 1 cup ditalini pasta
- Salt & pepper, to taste
- Finely chopped parsley, optional
- Grated parmesan, optional

Instructions

1. Heat a large dutch oven or a stockpot over medium heat.
2. Add in the ground beef, onion, minced garlic, carrots, and celery, seasoned with salt and pepper, and cook until no longer pink (about 5 minutes). Drain the grease into a can.
3. Add in the kidney beans, white beans, tomato sauce, diced tomatoes, chicken broth, oregano, and thyme leaves into the pot. Stir to combine.
4. Once the liquid starts to boil, add in the pasta.
5. Reduce the heat and cook for 10 minutes, or until the pasta is done.
6. Serve with chopped parsley and grated parmesan, if desired.

9. Chili Pumpkin

Prep Time: 5 Minutes

Cook Time: 25 Minutes

Serves: 5

Ingredients

- 1lb. extra-lean ground beef
- 1cup chopped onion
- 1cup chopped yellow bell pepper
- 3cloves garlic, minced
- 2cups water
- 115-oz. can pumpkin
- 115-oz. can no-salt-added pinto beans or black beans, rinsed and drained
- 114.5-oz can no-salt-added fire-roasted diced tomatoes, undrained
- 18-oz. can tomato sauce
- 14-oz. can diced green chiles, undrained
- 1Tbsp packed brown sugar
- 1Tbsp chili powder
- 2tsp unsweetened cocoa powder
- 2tsp dried oregano, crushed

- 1/2 tsp ground cinnamon
- 3/4 tsp salt
- Plain fat-free Greek yogurt
- Chopped fresh cilantro and finely chopped onion

Instructions

1. In a 4- to 5-quart Dutch oven, cook beef, onion, bell pepper, and garlic over medium until beef is browned, stirring occasionally.
2. Stir in the water, pumpkin, beans, tomatoes, tomato sauce, green chiles, brown sugar, chili powder, cocoa powder, oregano, cinnamon, and salt. Bring to boiling; reduce heat. Simmer 30 to 45 minutes or until desired thickness, stirring occasionally. Top each serving with yogurt and sprinkle with cilantro and onion.

10. Warm Goat Cheese Salad

Prep Time: 5 Minutes

Cook Time: 25 Minutes

Serves:

Ingredients

- 1 log (4 oz) fresh goat cheese
- 1 cup bread crumbs
- 1 tsp dried thyme or Italian seasoning
- Salt and black pepper to taste
- 1 egg, lightly beaten
- 1/4 cup walnuts
- 16 cups mixed greens or arugula (6-oz bag)
- Balsamic vinaigrette
- 1 pear, peeled, cored, and sliced

Instructions

1. Slice the goat cheese into four 1/2" disks (a piece of unflavored dental floss makes this job easy).
2. If the cheese crumbles, use your hands to form it back into disks.

3. Pour the bread crumbs onto a plate and toss with the thyme and a pinch each of salt and pepper.
4. Dip the goat cheese into the egg, then into the crumb mixture and turn to coat evenly.
5. Place the disks on a plate and into the freezer for 15 minutes to firm up.
6. Preheat the oven to 450°F.
7. Place the goat cheese on a baking sheet coated with non-stick cooking spray and bake for 10 minutes, until the cheese is soft and the crumbs are toasted.
8. Remove. While the oven is still hot, toast the walnuts for 5 minutes.
9. Toss the lettuce with the vinaigrette and pear. Divide among 4 cold plates. Top with the walnuts and goat cheese.

Fresh Goat Cheese:

1. Break free from the reliance on cheddar and mozzarella and discover some of the truly fantastic cheeses that too many serious eaters overlook. Fresh goat cheese has a tangy creaminess that makes it one of the most versatile in the dairy case, great for crumbling onto salads, spreading on sandwiches, or folding into warm pasta dishes. Our favorite goat cheeses are made by Cypress Grove Chevre and are available in supermarkets nationwide. An ounce has just 70 calories and 6 grams of fat, making it one of the healthiest cheeses you'll find.

LUNCH

11. Hot Ham and Cheese Sandwich with Chipotle Mayo

Prep Time: 25 Minutes

Cook Time: 55 Minutes

Serves: 4

Ingredients

For the mayo:
- 1/2 cup light mayonnaise
- 2 chipotle chiles in adobo sauce
- 1 Tbsp adobo sauce from chipotle peppers

For the sandwiches:
- 4 3/4-inch-thick slices sourdough bread
- 1 Tbsp butter, softened
- 8 oz thinly sliced low-sodium deli ham
- 4 ultra-thin slices pepper jack cheese
- Vegetable oil
- 1 tsp vinegar
- 4 large cold eggs

- salt
- Ground chipotle powder
- Microgreens or chopped fresh chives

Instructions
1. Preheat oven to 350°F. For the mayo, combine mayonnaise, chipotle chiles, and adobo sauce in a blender or food processor and blend until smooth.
2. For sandwiches, lightly butter both sides of the bread with softened butter. Toast one side of bread in an extra-large oven-proof skillet over medium heat until golden brown. Flip bread slices. While second side is toasting, spread top slice of bread with 1 tablespoon of the mayonnaise. Top with ham and cheese. Transfer pan to oven.
3. While sandwiches are heating, lightly oil the sides of a medium skillet or large saucepan. Fill pan half full with water. Add vinegar to water and bring to a boil.
4. Break 1 egg into a small dish. Carefully slide the egg into the simmering water, holding the lip of the dish as close to the water as possible. Repeat with three remaining eggs, adding them one at a time and spacing them so each egg has an equal amount of space surrounding it. Simmer for 3 to 5 minutes, or

until whites are completely set and yolks begin to thicken but are not hard.

5. Remove sandwiches from oven. Use a slotted spoon to remove eggs from water. Top each sandwich with an egg. Season lightly with salt and chipotle powder. Sprinkle with micro-greens and serve immediately.
6. Note: Refrigerate leftover mayo and use on sandwiches or add it as a topping for steamed or roasted vegetables.
7. Feeling devilish? Ditch the mayo in deviled eggs and swap for creamy avocado in the yolk mixture. This smarter preparation (avocado adds nutrients and healthy monounsaturated fats) makes a powerhouse midday snack or a crowd-pleasing appetizer.

12. Classic Herb Roast Chicken with Root Vegetables

Prep Time: 15 Minutes

Cook Time: 50 Minutes

Serves: 4

Ingredients

- 2 cloves garlic, minced
- 1 Tbsp finely chopped fresh rosemary (Almost any herb works here: thyme, parsley, oregano, basil, or sage)
- Zest and juice of 1 lemon
- 1 Tbsp olive oil
- 1 chicken (4 lb)
- Salt and black pepper to taste
- 1 large russet potato, sliced into 1/8" rounds
- 2 onions, quartered
- 4 large carrots, cut into large chunks

Instructions

1. Preheat the oven to 450°F. Mix the garlic, rosemary, lemon zest, and half of the olive oil.

2. Working on the chicken, gently separate the skin from the flesh at the bottom of the breast and spoon in half of the rosemary mixture; use your hands to spread it around as thoroughly as possible.
3. Spread the remaining half over the top of the chicken and then season with plenty of salt and pepper.
4. Mix the potato, onions, carrots, remaining olive oil, and a good pinch of salt and pepper.
5. Arrange the vegetables in the bottom of a roasting pan and place the chicken on top, breast side up.
6. Roast for 20 to 30 minutes, until the skin is lightly browned.
7. Reduce the oven temperature to 350°F and roast for another 30 minutes or so.
8. The chicken is done when the juices between the breast and the leg run clear and an instant-read thermometer inserted deep into the thigh reads 155°F.
9. Remove from the oven and allow to rest for 10 minutes before carving.
10. Serve with the vegetables.

Pre-salting

1. The question of when to salt meat is a subject of much debate in food science circles. Salt draws moisture out, which in theory can dry out a protein. But if you

leave it long enough, the moisture will be reabsorbed back into the meat, along with a big shot of seasoning. Rubbing the chicken all over with a teaspoon of kosher salt the night before allows the salt to penetrate all the way to the bone. If you want one way to combat dry, bland chicken, this is it.

13. Easy Cinnamon-Roasted Sweet Potato Salad with Wild Rice

Prep Time: 20 Minutes

Cook Time: 45 Minutes

Serves: 3

Ingredients

- Nonstick cooking spray
- 12 oz sweet potato, scrubbed and cut into 1/2-inch pieces
- 1 medium red or yellow onion, sliced into wedges
- 4 Tbsp olive oil
- 1 tsp salt
- 1/2 tsp black pepper
- 1/4 tsp ground cinnamon
- 2 Tbsp rice wine vinegar
- 1 Tbsp curry powder
- 2 tsp honey
- 1/2 tsp salt
- 1/4 tsp black pepper
- 2 cups cooked wild rice
- 4 oz cooked chicken, shredded
- 1/4 cup golden or regular raisins

- 2 medium carrots, shaved
- 1/4 cup snipped fresh cilantro

Instructions

1. Preheat oven to 400°F. Line a baking sheet with foil, and coat with cooking spray.
2. In a medium bowl, combine sweet potato, onion, 1 Tbsp oil, 1/2 tsp salt, 1/4 tsp pepper, and cinnamon; toss to coat. Transfer potato mixture to prepared baking sheet. Roast about 20 minutes or until tender.
3. Meanwhile, in a small bowl, combine remaining 3 Tbsp oil, vinegar, curry powder, honey, the remaining 1/2 tsp salt, and the remaining 1/4 tsp pepper. Whisk until smooth.
4. Divide rice among four pint jars. Top with roasted potatoes, chicken, raisins, and carrots. Drizzle with dressing and top with cilantro. Cover and chill up to 3 days.
5. Wild rice has nearly double the fiber and protein and fewer calories than brown rice.

14. Hearty Crock-Pot Beef Ragu

Prep Time: 23 Minutes

Cook Time: 60 Minutes

Serves: 5

Ingredients

- 1 lb. beef chuck
- 1 28 oz. can crushed tomatoes
- 1 6 oz. can tomato paste
- 1 cup carrots, peeled and diced
- 1 cup celery stalks, diced
- 2 garlic cloves, minced
- 1 medium onion, diced
- 1 teaspoon Italian seasoning
- 1 teaspoon salt
- 1/2 teaspoon pepper
- 1 cup of beef stock (or red wine)
- 1 bag/box of pappardelle pasta
- Shaved parmesan

Instructions

1. Season the beef with salt and pepper.

2. Add in seasoned beef, crushed tomatoes, tomato paste, carrots, celery, garlic cloves, onion, and Italian seasoning into a slow cooker.
3. Pour in the beef stock (or if you have some leftover red wine, use that).
4. Cook on low for 6 hours (8 hours max). If you cook for longer, the beef will get mushy, so be careful!
5. Right before serving, cook the pappardelle pasta in boiling water that has been lightly salted. Cook time varies based on packaging instructions.
6. Take the beef out and shred it with two forks. Place back in the sauce.
7. Serve beef ragu on prepared pappardelle pasta with shaved parmesan cheese.
8. Freeze this meal and save it for later! Add the seasoned beef, tomatoes, tomato paste, carrots, celery, garlic cloves, onion, and Italian seasoning into a gallon-size freezer bag. Make sure to defrost the meal in the refrigerator 24 hours before putting it into the slow cooker. Mix ingredients together so they are evenly distributed before turning on the slow cooker. Pour in the beef stock (or red wine) and follow the normal instructions from there.

15. Curry with Cauliflower and Butternut Squash Stir Fry

Prep Time: 23 Minutes

Cook Time: 60 Minutes

Serves: 5

Ingredients

- 1/2 Tbsp canola oil
- 1 medium onion, diced
- 1/2 Tbsp minced fresh ginger
- 2 cups cubed butternut squash (Carrots or potatoes would both be perfect substitutes for the squash, just in case butternut is not in season)
- 1 head cauliflower, cut into florets
- 1 can (14–16 oz) garbanzo beans (aka chickpeas), drained
- 1 jalapeño pepper, minced
- 1 Tbsp yellow curry powder
- 1 can (14 oz) diced tomatoes
- 1 can (14 oz) light coconut milk
- Juice of 1 lime
- Salt and black pepper to taste
- Chopped cilantro

Instructions

1. Heat the oil in a large sauté pan or pot over medium heat.
2. Add the onion and ginger and cook for about 2 minutes, until the onion is soft and translucent.
3. Add the squash, cauliflower, garbanzos, jalapeño, and curry powder. Cook for 2 minutes, until the curry powder is fragrant and coats the vegetables evenly.
4. Stir in the tomatoes and coconut milk and turn the heat down to low.
5. Simmer for 15 to 20 minutes, until the vegetables are tender.
6. Add the lime juice and season with salt and black pepper.
7. Serve garnished with the chopped cilantro.
8. At the heart of Indian curry powder is one of the world's most potent elixirs: curcumin, an antioxidant known to fight cancer, inflammation, bacteria, cholesterol, and a list of other maladies—large and small—too long to publish here. Curcumin resides in turmeric, the bright yellow spice that gives curries their characteristic hue. Don't limit the healing powers to recipes like this, though. Stir curry powder into yogurt for a vegetable dip, slip it into mayonnaise

for a powerful sandwich spread, or rub directly onto chicken or white fish before grilling.

16. Orecchiette with Broccoli Rabe

Prep Time: 25 Minutes

Cook Time: 40 Minutes

Serves: 4

Ingredients

- 1 bunch broccoli rabe, bottom 1" removed
- 10 oz orecchiette pasta
- 1/2 Tbsp olive oil
- 2 link sun cooked turkey or chicken sausage, casings removed
- 4 cloves garlic, minced
- 1/4 tsp red pepper flakes
- 3/4 cup low-sodium chicken stock
- Salt and black pepper to taste
- Pecorino Romano or Parmesan

Instructions

1. Bring a large pot of salted water to a boil. Drop in the broccoli rabe and cook for 3 minutes.
2. Use tongs to remove the greens and the chop into 1/2" pieces.

3. Return the water to a boil. Cook the pasta until al dente.
4. While the pasta cooks, heat the olive oil in a large skillet over medium heat.
5. Add the sausage and cook for about 5 minutes, until lightly browned, then add the garlic and pepper flakes and sauté for another 3 minutes.
6. Stir in the chopped broccoli rabe and chicken stock and lower the heat to a simmer.
7. Season with salt and pepper.
8. Drain the pasta and toss immediately into the pan with the sausage and greens.
9. Toss the pasta (if the mix looks dry, use a bit of the pasta cooking water to loosen it up).
10. Serve immediately with freshly grated cheese.
11. Calorie Cutting:
12. A serving size of pasta in Italy is about 6 ounces; here, many restaurant noodle bowls top 2 pounds. We've used more modest serving sizes for the noodles in the book's pasta recipes, but kept the sauce portions more substantial. That means the pasta-to-sauce ratio will skew toward the latter, which makes for a more satisfying meal for fewer calories.

17. The Best-Ever Healthy Lasagna

Prep Time: 15 Minutes

Cook Time: 45 Minutes

Serves: 8

Ingredients

- 1 Tbsp olive oil
- 3 links raw chicken sausage, casings removed
- 1 small onion, diced
- 2 cloves garlic, minced
- Pinch red pepper flakes
- 1 can (28 oz) crushed tomatoes
- Salt and black pepper to taste
- 1 1/2 cups low-fat ricotta (Barilla makes a good no-boil lasagna that is widely available.)
- 1/2 cup 2% milk
- 16 sheets no-boil lasagna noodles
- 16–20 fresh basil leaves
- 1 cup chopped fresh mozzarella

Instructions

1. Heat the olive oil in a large saucepan over medium heat.
2. Add the sausage and cook for about 3 minutes, until no longer pink.
3. Add the onion, garlic, and red pepper flakes and continue cooking for about 5 minutes, until the onion is soft and translucent.
4. Add the tomatoes and simmer for 15 minutes.
5. Season with salt and pepper.
6. Preheat the oven to 350 degrees Fahrenheit.
7. Combine the ricotta and milk in a mixing bowl.
8. In a 9" x 9" baking pan, lay down a layer of 4 noodles.
9. Cover with a quarter of the ricotta mixture and a quarter of the sausage mixture, then a few basil leaves and a quarter of the mozzarella.
10. Repeat three times to create a four-layer lasagna.
11. Cover with aluminum foil and bake for 25 minutes, until the cheese is melted and the pasta cooked through.
12. Remove the foil and increase the temperature to 450 degrees Fahrenheit.
13. Continue baking for about 10 minutes, until the top of the lasagna is nicely browned.

Other ways to layer your lasagna:

- Sautéed mushrooms and spinach (as many different types as you can find), béchamel, and goat cheese
- Turkey Bolognese and béchamel with a bit of grated Parmesan on top

18. Healthier Chicken Pot Pie

Prep Time: 20 Minutes

Cook Time: 55 Minutes

Serves: 4

Ingredients

- 2 Tbsp butter
- 1 onion, chopped
- 2 carrots, chopped
- 2 cloves garlic, minced
- 2 cups stemmed and quartered white or cremini mushrooms
- 2 cups frozen pearl onions
- 2 cups chopped cooked chicken (leftover or pulled from a store-bought rotisserie chicken)
- 1/4 cup flour
- 2 cups low-sodium chicken broth, warmed
- 1 cup 2% or whole milk
- 1/2 cup half-and-half
- 1 1/2 cups frozen peas
- Salt and black pepper to taste
- 1 sheet puff pastry, defrosted

- 2 egg whites, lightly beaten

Instructions
1. Heat the butter in a large sauté pan or pot over medium heat.
2. When it's melted, add the onion, carrots, and garlic and cook until the onion is translucent and the carrots begin to soften, about 5 minutes.
3. Add the mushrooms and pearl onions and cook, stirring occasionally, for another 5 minutes.
4. Stir in the chicken and the flour, using a wooden spoon to ensure the vegetables and meat are evenly coated with flour.
5. Slowly pour in the chicken broth, using a whisk to beat it in to help avoid clumping with the flour (having the broth warm or hot helps smooth out the sauce).
6. Once the broth is incorporated, add the milk and half-and-half and simmer for 10 to 15 minutes, until the sauce has thickened substantially and lightly clings to the vegetables and chicken. Stir in the peas. Season with salt and pepper.

7. Preheat the oven to 375°F. Cut the pastry into quarters. Roll out each piece on a floured surface to make a 6" square.
8. Divide the chicken mixture among 4 ovenproof bowls. Place a pastry square over the top of each bowl, and trim away the excess with a paring knife; pinch the dough around the edges of the bowl to secure it.
9. Brush the tops with the egg whites and bake until golden brown, about 25 minutes.
10. The bulk of the calories in pot pies comes from the butter-laden pastry that crowns the bowls. This recipe calls for puff pastry rolled extra thin to minimize the caloric impact, but to further reduce your fat intake, you can make two quick

Substitutions:

1. Instead of puff pastry, try a few layers of phyllo dough brushed with a bit of butter. Even then, it's still lighter and less caloric than puff pastry.
2. Replace the half-and-half with another 1/2 cup milk.

19. Beef Stew in Red Wine

Prep Time: 20 Minutes

Cook Time: 35 Minutes

Serves: 8

Ingredients

- 1 Tbsp canola oil
- 3 lb sirloin roast, brisket, or chuck, cut into 1" cubes
- 1 Tbsp flour
- Salt and black pepper to taste
- 2 medium onions, chopped
- 1 cup dry red wine, such as Pinot Noir or Cabernet Sauvignon
- 2 Tbsp tomato paste
- 2 cups chicken broth
- 3 bay leaves
- 8 branches fresh thyme (or 1 tsp dried)
- 6 medium red potatoes, cut into ½" pieces
- 3 medium carrots, peeled and chopped
- 2 cups frozen pearl onions
- 1 cup frozen peas
- Chopped fresh parsley or gremolata

Instructions

1. Heat ½ tablespoon of the oil in a large cast-iron skillet or sauté pan over medium-high heat. Combine the beef and flour in a bowl, season with salt and pepper, and toss to lightly coat the beef.
2. Working in two batches to avoid crowding the pan, sear the beef in the hot oil, turning occasionally, until nicely browned. Transfer to a slow cooker.
3. Add the remaining oil to the skillet.
4. Add the chopped onions and cook for about 5 minutes, until lightly browned.
5. Stir in the wine and tomato paste, scraping the bottom of the pan to free up any browned bits.
6. Pour the onion mixture over the beef, then add the broth, bay leaves, and thyme.
7. Set the slow cooker to high, cover, and cook for about 4 hours (or on low for 8 hours), until the beef is fork-tender.
8. An hour before serving, add the potatoes, carrots, and pearl onions.
9. Five minutes before serving, add the peas.
10. Discard the bay leaves and thyme branches and season with salt and black pepper.

11. Serve garnished with parsley or gremolata if you like.
12. While classic beef stew comes with no splashy garnishes, intense meaty dishes like this one are best when finished with a fresh, contrasting note. Cue gremolata, a combination of garlic, parsley, and lemon used to garnish bold Italian dishes like osso buco. The combination also works perfectly on top of grilled steak, roast chicken, and even pasta. To make, combine 2 tablespoons minced garlic with ½ cup minced fresh parsley and 1 tablespoon grated lemon zest.

20. Turkey Meatloaf

Prep Time: 22 Minutes

Cook Time: 45 Minutes

Serves: 4

Ingredients

For the turkey meatloaf:
- 1 small onion, peeled and quartered
- ½ red bell pepper, stemmed and quartered
- 1 small carrot, peeled and roughly chopped
- 2 cloves garlic, peeled
- 1 ½ lb ground turkey
- ½ cup bread crumbs
- ¼ cup low-sodium chicken stock
- 1 egg, beaten
- 1 Tbsp Worcestershire
- 1 Tbsp low-sodium soy sauce
- ½ tsp dried thyme
- ½ tsp salt
- ½ tsp black pepper

For the glaze:

- ½ cup ketchup
- 2 Tbsp brown sugar
- 2 Tbsp low-sodium soy sauce
- 2 Tbsp apple cider vinegar

Instructions
1. Preheat the oven to 325°F.
2. Combine the onion, bell pepper, carrot, and garlic in a food processor and pulse until finely minced. (If you don't have a food processor, you can do this by hand.)
3. Combine the vegetables with the turkey, bread crumbs, stock, egg, Worcestershire, soy sauce, thyme, and salt and black pepper in a large mixing bowl.
4. Gently mix until all of the ingredients are evenly distributed.
5. Dump the meatloaf mixture into a 13" x 9" baking dish and use your hands to form a loaf roughly 9" long and 6" wide.
6. Mix the glaze ingredients together and spread over the meatloaf.
7. Bake for 1 hour, until the glaze has turned a deep shade of red and an instant-read thermometer inserted into the center of the loaf registers 160°F.

8. There are more than a few ways to reinvent meatloaf the next day (topped with a fried egg, covered with sautéed peppers and onions), but for our money, the best bet is still a thick meatloaf sandwich. Gently sauté onions until nicely caramelized while reheating the meatloaf in a 325°F oven with a thin slice of smoked gouda, and serve it all on a toasted bun. It's worth making this recipe for the sandwich alone.

DINNERS

21. Creamy Mushroom Chicken

Prep Time: 35 Minutes

Cook Time: 50 Minutes

Serves: 4

Ingredients

- 1 Tbsp olive oil, plus more if needed
- 4 small boneless skinless chicken breasts (6 oz each)
- Salt and black pepper to taste
- 1 medium shallot, minced
- 3 cloves garlic, minced
- 8 oz cremini mushrooms, sliced
- ¼ cup sherry (In a pinch, sweet, fortified wines like Madeira or Marsala will work in place of the sherry.)
- ¼ cup dried mushrooms (porcini, chanterelle, shiitake), soaked in ½ cup warm water for 15 minutes
- ½ cup low-sodium chicken stock
- ¼ cup half-and-half
- ¼ cup Greek yogurt

Instructions

1. Heat the olive oil over high heat in a large sauté pan.
2. Season the chicken all over with salt and black pepper.
3. Add the chicken to the pan and sear for about 3 minutes, until a nice deep brown crust develops on the bottom sides.
4. Flip and continue to cook for 3 minutes longer, until the other sides are also nicely browned.
5. Remove to a plate.
6. If the pan is dry after cooking the chicken, add a thin film of olive oil.
7. Add the shallot, garlic, and cremini mushrooms to the pan and sauté for about 3 minutes, until the mushrooms are lightly browned.
8. Season with salt and black pepper.
9. Add the sherry and cook for 1 minute, using a spatula or wooden spoon to scrape loose any browned bits from the bottom of the pan.
10. Add the dried mushrooms (and soaking liquid), chicken stock, and half-and-half.
11. Turn the heat down to low and return the chicken to the pan.

12. Continue cooking for 8 to 10 minutes, until the liquid reduces by half and the chicken is cooked through.
13. Add the yogurt and stir to create a smooth, uniform sauce.
14. Divide the chicken among 4 plates and top with the mushroom sauce.

22. Zucchini Carbonara with Bacon

Prep Time: 15 Minutes

Cook Time: 55 Minutes

Serves: 4

Ingredients

- 10 oz spaghetti
- 6 strips bacon, cut into ½" pieces
- 1 medium yellow onion, diced
- 1 large zucchini, sliced into thin ribbons
- 2 cloves garlic, sliced
- Salt and black pepper to taste
- 2 eggs
- Pecorino or Parmesan for grating
- 1 handful chopped fresh parsley

Instructions

1. Bring a large pot of salted water to a boil.
2. Add the pasta and cook until al dente (usually about 30 seconds to a minute less than the package instructions recommend).

3. While the pasta cooks, heat a large sauté pan over medium heat.
4. Add the bacon and cook until crispy, about 5 minutes.
5. Transfer the bacon to a plate lined with paper towels.
6. Discard all but a thin film of the fat from the pan.
7. Add the onion, zucchini, and garlic and cook for 5 to 7 minutes, until soft and lightly browned.
8. Stir back in the bacon and season with a bit of salt and plenty of coarse black pepper.
9. Drain the pasta, using a coffee cup to save a few ounces of the cooking water.
10. Add the pasta directly to the sauté pan and toss to coat.
11. Stir in enough of the pasta water so that a thin layer of moisture clings to the noodles.
12. Remove from the heat and crack the two eggs directly into the pasta, using tongs or two forks to toss for even distribution.
13. Divide the pasta among four warm bowls or plates and top with grated cheese and parsley.

23. Flavorful Basque Chicken

Prep Time: 25 Minutes

Cook Time: 30 Minutes

Serves: 4

Ingredients

- 1 Tbsp olive oil
- 4 bone-in, skin-on chicken breasts
- Salt and black pepper to taste
- 1 link Spanish chorizo, sliced into 1/4"-thick coins
- 1 bottle (12 oz) porter, stout, or other dark beer
- 1 1/2 cups low-sodium chicken stock
- 2 Tbsp sherry vinegar or red wine vinegar
- 1 large onion, quartered
- 1 red bell pepper, chopped
- 8 cloves garlic, peeled
- 1 tsp smoked paprika
- 1/2 tsp cumin
- 2 bay leaves
- 4 cups baby spinach (optional)

Instructions
1. Heat the olive oil in a large cast-iron skillet or sauté pan over medium-high heat.
2. Season the chicken all over with salt and black pepper and cook the pieces until browned on all sides, about 7 minutes.
3. Add the chorizo and continue cooking for another 2 minutes, until the chorizo has browned as well.
4. Transfer the meat to the slow cooker.
5. Pour the beer into the skillet, scraping the bottom to loosen any brown bits.
6. Add to the slow cooker, along with the stock, vinegar, onion, bell pepper, garlic, paprika, cumin, and bay leaves and cook on low for 4 hours.
7. If using spinach, add it 10 minutes before serving, giving it enough time to cook down in the warm braising liquid.
8. Before serving, discard the bay leaves and taste and adjust the seasoning with salt and black pepper.
9. Serve in wide shallow bowls with a ladle of the braising liquid poured over the top.

24. Spicy Macaroni and Cheese with Jalapeños and Prosciutto

Prep Time: 30 Minutes

Cook Time: 55 Minutes

Serves: 4

Ingredients

- 2 Tbsp butter
- 1/2 yellow onion, minced
- 2 Tbsp flour
- 3 cups milk
- 2 cups shredded extra-sharp Cheddar
- Salt and black pepper to taste
- 1 lb elbow macaroni, penne, or shells
- 1/4 cup chopped pickled jalapeños
- 2 oz prosciutto or ham, cut into thin strips
- 1/2 cup panko bread crumbs
- 1/4 cup grated Parmesan

Instructions

1. Preheat the oven to 375°F.
2. Melt the butter in a large saucepan over medium heat. Add the onion and cook until soft and translucent (but

not browned), about 3 minutes. Add the flour and stir to incorporate into the butter.

3. Pour in the milk a few tablespoons at a time, using a whisk to incorporate the flour and prevent lumps from forming.
4. When all the milk has been added, allow the sauce to simmer for 10 minutes, until it begins to thicken. Stir in the cheese and season with salt and pepper.
5. Cook the pasta according to the package instructions until al dente, drain, and return to the pot. Add the cheese sauce, jalapeños, and prosciutto and stir to fully incorporate.
6. Divide the mixture among 6 individual crocks or pour into a large baking dish. Top with the bread crumbs and sprinkle with the Parmesan.
7. Bake for 10 minutes. Turn on the broiler and broil until the bread crumbs are golden brown and crispy, about another 3 minutes.
8. Classic Cheddar-based mac and cheese is tough to beat, but besides having high calorie and fat counts, it also provides little redeeming nutrition. Boost the health profile (and the hunger-squashing potential) of your mac and cheese by adding any of the following to the pasta when you toss it with the cheese sauce.

- 1 cup caramelized onions
- 2 cups roughly chopped or cherry tomatoes
- 6 oz grilled chicken and 1 cup sautéed mushrooms
- 2 cups chopped steamed or sautéed broccoli

25. Paleo Turkey Bolognese with Garlic Spaghetti Squash

Prep Time: 25 Minutes

Cook Time: 40 Minutes

Serves: 4

Ingredients

- 1 medium spaghetti squash (2 1/2 to 3 pounds)
- 1 bulb garlic
- 3 Tbsp extra-virgin olive oil
- 1 pound ground turkey
- 1 cup finely chopped carrots (2)
- 1/2 cup finely chopped onion (1 medium)
- 1/2 cup finely chopped celery (1 stalk)
- 4 cloves garlic, minced
- 3 Tbsp tomato paste
- 1/2 cup dry red wine
- 1 (28-ounce) can crushed tomatoes
- 1 tsp dried oregano, crushed
- 1 tsp dried basil, crushed
- 1 tsp fennel seeds, lightly crushed
- 3/4 tsp salt, divided

- 3/4 tsp pepper, divided
- 1/2 cup reduced-sodium chicken broth

Instructions

1. Preheat oven to 375°F. Halve the squash lengthwise and scrape out the seeds. Place squash halves, cut sides down, in a large baking dish. Prick skin all over with a fork. Cut 1/2 inch off the top of the head of garlic. Place, cut end up, in the baking dish with squash. Drizzle with 1 tablespoon olive oil. Bake 35 to 45 minutes or until squash and garlic are tender.
2. While squash is baking, heat 1 tablespoon of the oil in a large pot over medium heat. Add turkey, carrots, onion, celery, and garlic. Cook until turkey is cooked through and vegetables are tender, stirring with a wooden spoon to break up meat.
3. Add tomato paste; cook and stir for 1 minute. Add red wine; cook and stir for 1 minute. Stir in tomatoes, oregano, basil, fennel, and 1/2 teaspoon each salt and pepper. Add broth and bring to boiling. Reduce heat and simmer, uncovered, 30 minutes or until desired consistency.
4. Using a fork, remove and shred flesh from each squash half; transfer to a bowl and cover to keep

warm. When garlic is cool enough to handle, squeeze bulb from bottom to pop out the cloves into a small bowl. Add remaining 1 tablespoon oil to garlic. Mash with a fork. Stir mashed garlic into spaghetti squash and season with remaining 1/4 teaspoon salt and pepper.

5. Serve meat sauce over spaghetti squash.

26. Tandoori Chicken Legs and Roasted Cauliflower

Prep Time: 25 Minutes

Cook Time: 40 Minutes

Serves: 3

Ingredients

- 1 lemon
- 2 chicken hindquarters or 4 chicken legs
- 1/2 cup plain whole-milk yogurt
- 1 Tbsp grated fresh ginger
- 3 cloves garlic, minced
- 1 Tbsp plus 1 tsp garam masala
- 1/2 tsp chili powder
- 1 tsp sea salt
- 2 Tbsp coconut oil or ghee, melted
- 2 cups cauliflower florets
- 2 Tbsp coarsely chopped pecans
- 1 Tbsp chopped fresh basil

Instructions

1. Season and cook the chicken. Zest and juice lemon. Place a resealable plastic bag in a large bowl. Add 1/2

teaspoon lemon zest, 2 tablespoons lemon juice, the yogurt, ginger, 2 cloves garlic, 1 tablespoon garam masala, the chili powder, and 1/2 teaspoon salt to bag. With a knife, make three slashes on top of chicken pieces; place chicken in bag and seal. (Slashing the chicken legs with a knife will allow all the zesty flavors of the marinade to penetrate the meat.) Gently massage bag to mix. Refrigerate overnight, turning the bag over occasionally. Preheat oven to 400 °F. Remove chicken from marinade (pieces will still be coated) and place on one end of a baking sheet. Roast 15 minutes.

2. Prep and roast the cauliflower. In a large bowl, combine 1 teaspoon lemon zest, 1 tablespoon lemon juice, and the remaining garlic, garam masala, and salt. Stir in coconut oil. Add cauliflower and stir until well coated. Remove baking sheet from oven; add cauliflower mixture to the other end, spreading into a single layer. Roast 30 minutes more or until chicken is no longer pink inside and cauliflower is tender and browned around edges. Add pecans to cauliflower for the last 5 minutes of roasting time. Remove from oven and toss cauliflower mixture with basil. Serve with chicken.

27. Pumpkin Version of Pad Thai

Prep Time: 15 Minutes

Cook Time: 36 Minutes

Serves: 5

Ingredients

- 6 oz. dry brown rice noodles
- 1/2 cup canned pumpkin
- 1/2 cup water
- 2 tbsp rice vinegar
- 1 tbsp packed brown sugar
- 1 tbsp creamy peanut butter
- 1 tbsp Asian chili sauce with garlic
- 2 cups shredded green and/or red cabbage
- 2 cups shredded cooked chicken
- 1 cup cooked shelled edamame
- 1/2 cup fresh cilantro leaves
- 1/4 cup sliced green onions
- 2 tbsp chopped unsalted peanuts
- crushed red pepper
- lime wedges

Instructions
1. Place noodles in a large bowl. Add enough boiling water to cover. Let stand according to package directions or until softened but still slightly chewy, stirring occasionally. Drain; snip noodles into shorter lengths.
2. For the sauce, in a bowl stir together pumpkin, the water, vinegar, brown sugar, peanut sauce, and chili sauce. Transfer sauce to four small cups.
3. In four bowls, arrange noodles, cabbage, chicken, edamame, and cilantro. Sprinkle with green onions, peanuts, and crushed red pepper. Nestle sauce cups into bowls. Serve with lime wedges.

28. Paleo BBQ Pork Shepherd's Pie with Sweet Potato Topping

Prep Time: 10 Minutes

Cook Time: 45 Minutes

Serves: 5

Ingredients

- 3 medium sweet potatoes (about 12 ounces)
- 2 Tbsp ghee
- 1/4 cup unsweetened plain almond milk
- 1/2 tsp salt, divided
- 1/2 tsp smoked paprika, plus additional for garnishing
- 1 pound ground pork
- 1/2 cup thinly sliced celery
- 1 cup frozen chopped onion and green sweet pepper blend
- 2 cups chopped fresh kale
- 3/4 cup paleo-compliant barbecue sauce
- 1/2 tsp ground cumin
- Chopped fresh parsley

Instructions
1. Preheat the oven to 425°F. Pierce the sweet potatoes with a fork in 5 to 6 places. Place on a microwavable plate and cook on high 5 to 8 minutes or until tender, rotating halfway through cook time; set aside to cool slightly. When cool enough to handle, peel and place in a mixing bowl. Mash with ghee, almond milk, 1/4 teaspoon salt, and smoked paprika until creamy.
2. Meanwhile, cook pork, celery, and onion and sweet pepper blend in a skillet over medium heat until meat is browned and vegetables are tender. Drain fat. Add kale, barbecue sauce, cumin, and remaining 1/4 teaspoon salt to skillet. Cook 1 to 2 minutes or until heated through. Transfer mixture to a 1 1/2-quart casserole or baking dish.
3. Spread sweet potato mixture over the pork mixture. Bake, uncovered, 10 minutes or until heated through and sweet potatoes are slightly browned.
4. Sprinkle with additional smoked paprika and chopped parsley.
5. How do you pick out a truly sweet tater? Look for firm skin that is even in tone and smooth to the touch. Typically, those with richer color are also richer in the awesome antioxidant beta-carotene.

29. Low-Calorie Braised Brisket with Horseradish

Prep Time: 25 Minutes

Cook Time: 55 Minutes

Serves: 4

Ingredients

- 1 Tbsp olive oil
- 3 lb brisket (preferably with a thin fat cap still attached)
- Salt and black pepper to taste
- 1 bottle (12 oz) dark beer
- 2 cups low-sodium chicken stock
- 2 Tbsp tomato paste
- 2 large yellow onions, quartered
- 1 bunch carrots, peeled
- 8 cloves garlic, peeled
- 2 bay leaves
- ¼ cup 2% Greek yogurt
- 2 Tbsp chopped fresh parsley
- 1 Tbsp prepared horseradish

Insructions

1. Heat the olive oil in a large cast-iron skillet or sauté pan.
2. Season the brisket all over with salt and black pepper.
3. Sear in the pan for about 7 minutes, until all sides are nicely browned.
4. Place in a slow cooker.
5. Add the beer to the pan and scrape up any browned bits. Pour over the brisket.
6. Add the stock, tomato paste, onions, carrots, garlic, and bay leaves to the slow cooker.
7. Cover and cook on high for 4 hours (or on low for up to 8 hours), until the brisket is very tender.
8. Combine the yogurt, parsley, and horseradish in a mixing bowl.
9. Remove the brisket from the cooker and slice into thin pieces. Discard the bay leaves.
10. Serve the brisket in a shallow, wide bowl with the onions, carrots, and a bit of broth poured over the top.
11. Garnish each serving with a scoop of the horseradish cream.
12. Leftover Love
13. Three ways to turn extra brisket into a next-day bounty:

- Brisket French Dip: Slice the brisket thinly, top with caramelized onions and Swiss. Serve with a warm cup of the braising liquid.
- Corned Beef Hash: Cook diced potatoes and onions in a pan until soft, then stir in shredded brisket, Dijon mustard, Worcestershire, and some of the leftover braising liquid.
- Brisket Nachos: Shred the meat, then use it to top tortilla chips along with pepper-Jack cheese, pinto beans, sliced jalapeños, and salsa verde.

30. Easy Chicken and Dumplings

Prep Time: 35 Minutes

Cook Time: 50 Minutes

Serves: 4

Ingredients

- 2 Tbsp butter
- 4 medium carrots, diced
- 1 medium onion, diced
- 3 Tbsp plus 2/3 cup flour
- 1/2 tsp dried thyme
- 4 cups low-sodium chicken stock
- 1 lb boneless, skinless chicken thighs
- Salt and black pepper to taste
- 1 1/2 tsp baking powder
- 1 tsp chopped fresh rosemary
- 1/2 cup 2% milk
- 1/2 cup frozen peas

Instructions

1. Heat the butter in a pot or large saucepan over medium heat.
2. Add the carrots and onions and cook for about 5 minutes, until softened.
3. Add the 3 tablespoons flour and the thyme, stirring so that the vegetables are evenly coated.
4. Slowly add the stock, whisking to prevent lumps from forming. Bring to a gentle simmer.
5. Season the chicken thighs with salt and black pepper and add to the pot, submerging them in the stock.
6. Poach the chicken for about 8 minutes, until just cooked through.
7. Remove to a cutting board to rest.
8. Combine the remaining 2/3 cup flour with the baking powder, rosemary, 1/4 teaspoon salt, and lots of black pepper.
9. Add the milk and gently stir until the dough just comes together.
10. Form loosely into 8 dumplings and drop them directly into the soup.
11. Cover the pot and cook over low heat for 10 minutes, until the dumplings have firmed up.

12. Shred the reserved chicken.
13. Add to the pot, along with the peas, stirring carefully so as not to break up the dumplings.
14. Heat through for 1 minute before serving.

Printed in Great Britain
by Amazon